Diabetes No More
Step By Step Guide to End Diabetes

Table of Contents

About the Book 2

About the Author 3

Introduction 4

Chapter 1 – Understanding Diabetes 5

    What is Diabetes? 5

    Types of Diabetes 6

    What Causes Diabetes? 11

    What Are the Symptoms Associated with Diabetes? 13

    Treatment for Diabetes – What's the Plan? 15

Chapter 2 – Diabetes & Eating – What's Right & Wrong? 18

    Choosing Healthy Foods 18

    Understanding Carbohydrates 19

    Learn the Diabetes Super Foods 21

    Limit Sugar & Desserts 22

    Choose the Right Fats 23

    Artifical Sweeteners – Are They Really Better? 24

    What to Eat – Summary 25

    What to Avoid - Summary 25

Chapter 3 – Diabetic Meal Plan 27

    The Basics 27

    Meal Plan Examples 28

Chapter 4 – Diabetic Diet Q&A 42

    Preventing Diabetes with Diabetic Diet – Can it be done? 42

    Diabetic Diet for the Whole Family – Is it safe? 42

    Diabetic Diet for Teens & Picky Eaters – Is there such a thing? 43

    Diabetic Meal Plan on the Go – What if I travel a lot? 44

    Combining Gluten Free & Diabetic Meals 44

    What is the Difference Between the Diabetic Diet & the Glycemic Index Diet? 45

    What Role Does Exercise Play in Diabetes Management? 46

About the Book

This book is an outline of diabetes as a whole, including the different types, causes, treatment methods, prevention tips and most important of all, a diabetic meal plan to ensure the body is getting everything it needs and nothing it doesn't. Chapter 1 focuses on understanding diabetes and learning the variances between the different types: Type 1, Type 2, gestational, prediabetes and diabetes insipidus. You will gain an understanding of the causes, the symptoms, the treatment methods and what you can do to help prevent diabetes, which is the 7th leading cause of death in the United States.

You will then get into Chapter 2, where you will learn about what foods you should and should not eat if you have been diagnosed with diabetes. You will discover the different types of carbohydrates, learn to evaluate the difference between good fats and bad fats and learn the truth about whether or not artificial sweeteners are beneficial. You will also learn how to choose the right foods to put on your plate, how to dish up the appropriate portion sizes, and some appropriate portion sizes, and how to prepare healthy snacks.

Once you take in all the background information related to diabetes and healthy diabetic eating, you can dive into Chapter 3, where there are specific meal plan suggestions laid out for you in easy to understand charts. Each meal can be modified to meet your tastes, while offering you examples of how to begin planning a specific diabetic diet based upon the guidelines in Chapter 2. Once you've finished reading this chapter, you will be ready to head to the grocery store to begin preparing healthy balanced meals.

Finally, Chapter 4 answers countless other questions you may have about diabetes, including topics about traveling while managing diabetes to whether or not a diabetic diet is right for the entire family. You will also discover how to incorporate more fruits and vegetables into a picky teenager's diabetic diet plan as well. Lastly, you will read information on exercise and the glycemic index, making it easy to find all the information you need to help manage your diabetes successfully.

The book has been written with love and with no intention of confusing you or making you feel inadequate when it comes to what you do and don't know about diabetes. It is, however, determined to not only help you gain a deeper understanding of the disease, but to help you learn to plan accordingly no matter what the situation. This will ensure that you have the means to get your diabetes under control, so that you can begin living the healthy, active life you have always dreamed of!

About the Author

Although not a physician, the author, Lisa K. Randalls, has an extensive background in knowledge of diabetes. Lisa has studied diabetes intently, including the types, causes, symptoms and treatment methods used to control the disease. Her main focus when beginning research into diabetes was to determine proper health and nutrition for herself and a family member. Lisa K. Randalls developed Type 1 diabetes at an early age, and her family member developed Type 2 diabetes later in life due to life struggles that caused depression and poor eating choices, leading to a lack of physical activity and obesity.

With a passion for discovering the truth about diabetes, and knowing the importance of sharing that information with others to help prevent future diagnoses of diabetes, particularly in the youth across America, Lisa K. Randalls has brought this book to life. She is determined to spread the word about this overwhelming disease, informing everyone how important it is to take care of themselves and their loved ones who have been diagnosed with this disease.

Although her disease could not be prevented, it saddens her to know that each day more and more cases of Type 2 diabetes – the preventable type – are being diagnosed due to childhood obesity and a lack of knowledge, power and self-control. Children learn from their parents their habits – good and bad. Unfortunately, some of these bad habits have led to overwhelming numbers in obesity in America, thus leading to Type 2 diabetes, something that can so simply be prevented by changing the way America eats and increasing their physical activity.

Through her own trials and tribulations with the disease, learning to manage the ins and outs of diabetes from many different angles, she knows how difficult it can be for those who are newly diagnosed. Learning what to eat and what not to eat can be overwhelming by itself, let alone managing the medications needed to treat the disease. She gives anyone who has been diagnosed with diabetes the strength and the courage to hang in there. It will get better, and you will soon understand, as she has finally come to realize that managing her condition can be simple.

Introduction

Whether or not they know the ins and outs of diabetes, most Americans have heard the term at some point or other in their life. In fact, the American Diabetes Association (ADA) believes that there are approximately 16 to 26 million Americans coping with diabetes. Even with more than 700,000 newly diagnosed cases of diabetes each year, research has found that more than 5 million individuals do not even know they have the disease.

In the past, diabetes has been thought of as a disease for older adults, but due to the overwhelming childhood obesity in this nation, it has become one of the most common medical issues for the younger generations as well. In fact, it has been discovered that more than 120,000 children and teens under the age of 18 have diabetes, and the U.S. Department of Health and Human Services has declared it the 7th leading cause of death for Americans no matter their age.

All types of diabetes are treatable or manageable. Unfortunately, what shouldn't be happening is the diagnosis of so many cases of diabetes in America, especially since it is a preventable disease just by changing eating habits and involving yourself in exercise or physical activity. Fortunately, if a person has been diagnosed with certain forms of preventable diabetes, it is possible for them to reverse the effects and cure themselves from having diabetes any longer. But for now, the first step for each newly diagnosed case of diabetes – and those who have known for a while – is to learn how to manage their disease through diet and exercise – with the help of medications along the way.

Chapter 1 – Understanding Diabetes

Gaining control of diabetes begins with understanding the disease. While it is not necessary to become a diabetes expert, it is important that a person with diabetes understands what it is, why it happens, what the different types are and what treatment methods are available. Having knowledge of an overview of diabetes is a good starting point to a new, healthier you.

What is Diabetes?

First and foremost, diabetes mellitus, known more commonly as diabetes, is actually a group of diseases that cause high blood glucose (sugar) levels as a result of the body's inability to produce and/or use insulin properly. This leads to improper ways of the body using digested food for energy, normal daily functions and in some cases, alters growth. When food is consumed, it is broken down during the digestive process and becomes a simple sugar known as glucose.

Glucose serves as the body's primary source of fuel and energy. During the digestive process, when the body works properly, glucose gets absorbed into the bloodstream where the body converts it into usable energy, using insulin, which is made by the pancreas. The job of the pancreas is to regulate production of insulin and move glucose from the blood into the cells where it is needed.

Unfortunately, this is not the case with diabetic individuals. The pancreas of an individual with diabetes fails to produce insulin, or produces insufficient amounts of insulin, wherein the body does not have enough cells to respond to the lack of insulin produced. In the end, glucose builds up in the blood, overflows to the urine and is passed out of the body. While this may not seem like a big deal, it is. In fact, by passing needed glucose through the urine, the body is losing important nutrients that serve as fuel for every day functions.

You may be thinking – but the body is producing glucose, what's the problem. True, the body is produce the glucose, as that occurs by digesting the foods you eat. However, where the problem lies is in the fact that the body is not producing enough insulin to properly transport the glucose from the blood and into the cells to be put to good use. In general, diabetes is the excess glucose that remains in the blood as opposed to moving into the cells, causing high blood sugar levels, and often leading to more severe complications.

Types of Diabetes

Many have heard of Type 1 diabetes and Type 2 diabetes. However, there are many different types of diabetes that can affect different individuals at different times in life, including gestational diabetes, prediabetes and diabetes insipidus. While they are all similar in that every type of diabetes affects blood sugar levels, they come about due to different causes and sometimes have different treatment options and/or prevention methods.

Type 1 Diabetes

The first type of diabetes to be aware of is Type 1 diabetes, which results when the body's immune system begins destroying the cells located in the pancreas, known as beta cells, that produce insulin. In a person without diabetes, the body's immune system fights off viruses and/or bacterial infection. However, this is not so in an individual with Type 1 diabetes. In fact, in a Type 1 diabetic the immune system attacks the body's own cells, which results in a deficiency of the hormone that produces insulin.

Because the main role of insulin is to move nutrients – particularly sugar – into the body's cells in order to convert it into needed energy, this negatively impacts the body's health and ability to function. Furthermore, sugar in the blood decreases when it enters the cells, which in a non-diabetic individual, alerts the pancreas to reduce the amount of insulin it creates in order to prevent hypoglycemia – low blood sugar levels. However, because the beta cells get destroyed in an individual with Type 1 diabetes, this process goes into disarray.

Due to a lack of insulin to push the sugar into the cells, the sugar builds up in the blood and the cells in the body lack vital nutrients, causing the body to find other means of providing energy for bodily functions. This is what is referred to as high blood sugar and can result in weight loss, dehydration, diabetic ketoacidosis – breakdown of fact cells that causes acid build up – and damages to the other parts of the body. This can include damaged blood vessels in the eyes, and damage to the kidneys and heart, which can lead to hardening of the arteries – atherosclerosis. Atherosclerosis is a major risk factor for developing heart disease and/or having heart attacks and strokes.

Typically, Type 1 diabetes is diagnosed in the early years of life, prior to age 20, especially because it is a body malfunction. However, it is a disease that can occur at any time. While diabetes is a very prevalent disease among Americans, only about 5% of individuals diagnosed with diabetes have Type 1. This type of diabetes equally affects men and women, and is more often diagnosed in Caucasians rather than African Americans.

Type 2 Diabetes

Type 2 diabetes is the second type of diabetes to learn about, yet the most commonly diagnosed form of the disease. In fact, Type 2 diabetes affects about 90% - 95% of Americans diagnosed with diabetes, and is often referred to as non-insulin dependent diabetes. This is because individuals with Type 2 diabetes, unlike those with Type 1 diabetes, have the ability to produce insulin. Unfortunately, two things occur in those with Type 2 diabetes, which result in the disease. One, for some reason the body is unable to make adequate use of the insulin produced. Two, although insulin is being produced, the pancreas simply does not produce enough. This results in a phenomenon known as insulin resistance, wherein insulin no longer has the ability to keep blood sugar levels within normal limits.

As with individuals who have Type 1 diabetes, people with Type 2 diabetes experience the same situation where glucose cannot move into the body's cells where it should be. This, in turn, causes a buildup of sugar in the blood, resulting in damage to the nerves, the blood vessels in the eyes, the kidneys and the heart, where it once again begins to harden the arteries – atherosclerosis – putting the individual at an increased risk for heart attacks and strokes.

Because the extra amounts of sugar in the blood lead to increases in urination, diabetics are at an increased risk for dehydration. Dehydration can further lead to a condition known as hyperosmolar nonketotic diabetic coma, more commonly referred to as a diabetic coma, which is a life-threatening situation. This occurs when individuals with Type 2 diabetes become so severely dehydrated or ill that they are unable to take in necessary fluids that are being lost as a result of excessive urination. This makes having proper amounts of fluid intake – particularly water – so much more important for an individual with Type 2 diabetes, or any form of the disease that causes increases in urination.

Furthermore, it is sad, but true, to report that Type 2 diabetes is being diagnosed in children at much higher rates than in the past. Research has shown that approximately 186,000 young adults have been and are being diagnosed with both Type 1 and Type 2 diabetes, with the emphasis on Type 2 diabetes. It is important to realize that because a child's body is more insulin resistant that that of an adult, larger amounts of sugar/glucose build up in the bloodstream. While this is dangerous for an adult, it is even worse for a child and, over time, can cause heart disease, kidney failure and blindness, at much early ages in life.

Children who are overweight, particularly females with a family history of diabetes and are of certain descent – African-American, American Indian, Asian or Hispanic/Latino – are at an increased risk of developing Type 2 diabetes. However, the most important risk factor to be aware of is excess weight in children, particularly abdominal weight, which results from poor eating habits, decreased physical activity, habits inherited by family members and in rare cases, medical conditions or issues related to hormonal imbalances.

Aside from children who are affected by Type 2 diabetes, adults are at risk for the same complications as well. Overweight adults who are over the age of 45, have experienced gestational diabetes in the past or have a family member diagnosed with Type 2 diabetes are at a higher risk for developing the disease. Other risk factors include individuals who have been diagnosed with prediabetes, lack physical activity, have high triglyceride levels and/or low HDL (good) cholesterol or have been diagnosed with high blood pressure. Similar to the risks children face, adults of similar ethnic backgrounds are at increased risk as well.

Gestational Diabetes

Gestational diabetes is the third type of diabetes and affects approximately 4% of pregnant women, as a result of high blood sugar levels during pregnancy. Gestational diabetes develops because hormonal changes during pregnancy can cause glucose intolerance. Although this means that a woman's blood sugar levels are higher than when they are not pregnant, this does not mean they are high enough to be classified as having Type 1 or Type 2 diabetes, especially after giving birth.

However, this does not mean that the woman is not at risk for complications caused by the gestational diabetes. In fact, in the early stages of pregnancy – the first trimester - the growth of the fetus can be affected, resulting in possible birth defects of the brain and/or heart, as well as an increased chance of having a miscarriage.

In later stages of pregnancy – the second and third trimesters – gestational diabetes in the mother can cause nutritional overload for the growing baby, resulting in larger babies, a condition known as macrosomia. Having a large baby can cause complications during labor and delivery to both the mother and the baby. For instance, the mother may need to have a C-section delivery or if the baby is born vaginally, he/she may cause damage to their shoulders when coming through the birth canal.

Furthermore, if the fetus receives too much nutrition, it is possible that hyperinsulinemia can occur. This means that the baby's blood sugar levels can decrease drastically after birth as a result of no longer receiving high amounts of blood sugar from mother. Fortunately, with careful monitoring and following all of the physician's orders, a healthy baby can be delivered despite having gestational diabetes.

Pregnant women at an increased risk for developing gestational diabetes include those who are overweight prior to pregnancy, are of a specific ethnic background – Hispanic, African-American, Native American or Asian, have sugar in their urine, altered glucose tolerance, including fasting glucose tolerance, and a family member who has had diabetes, such as a sibling or parent.

In addition, other factors that lead to an increased risk of having gestational diabetes include having given birth to a large baby – over 9 pounds – prior to the current pregnancy, previously having gestational diabetes or having a condition known as polyhydramnios – too much amniotic fluid. Fortunately, most women are tested during early pregnancy by means of an oral glucose tolerance test and are able to begin management of the disease at an early stage.

Prediabetes

Surprisingly, there are approximately 79 million Americans over the age of 20 who have prediabetes, a condition in which blood sugar levels are high, but not so high that they qualify an individual for being diagnosed with the disease. Often known by other names, such as impaired glucose tolerance and/or impaired fasting glucose, prediabetes is a condition with no symptoms, but is present prior to the majority of diagnosed cases of Type 2 diabetes. Furthermore, doctors are beginning to realize the importance of discovering and diagnosing prediabetes in order to prevent other serious conditions, particularly diabetes, which can lead to conditions such as blood vessel and heart disease, as well as kidney and eye disease.

Individuals who should be examined for possibly having prediabetes include those who are 45 years old or older and have a body mass index (BMI) of 25 or more. Talking to a physician is important for any individual who has multiple risk factors for developing Type 2 diabetes. This can include a physically inactive lifestyle, personal history of gestational diabetes and family history of diabetes, to name a few. Combined, these risk factors could mean that a person has prediabetes, but due to lack of symptoms, is not aware of their condition.

There are three different types of blood tests used to determine whether or not an individual has prediabetes or any form of the disease. During a fasting plasma glucose test the patient fasts for a minimum of 8 hours prior to the blood sugar levels being measured. In an oral glucose tolerance test blood sugar levels are examined twice. First, the patient will be tested after a period of fasting. Secondly, they will be given a glucose beverage and then wait for two hours before being tested again. The final test used in diagnosing diabetes is the hemoglobin A1C test that can determine average blood sugar levels over the past 3-4 months. After each test, doctors are able to determine whether or not the blood sugar levels indicate impaired glucose tolerance, thus suggesting prediabetes, or in some cases an actual diagnosis of diabetes, typically Type 2.

Diabetes Insipidus

The fifth and final type of diabetes is diabetes insipidus, which is slightly different than diabetes mellitus. It should be noted that diabetes is a general term for a broad spectrum of diseases wherein urine production is increased. While other types of diabetes can, and do, increase urine production, extreme thirst and very high levels of urination come from diabetes insipidus.

This can be attributed to problems with the hormone known as antidiuretic hormone and/or its receptor. The antidiuretic hormone is created in the hypothalamus – a part of the brain – and stored in the pituitary gland – also located in the brain. When antidiuretic hormones are released, this causes the kidneys to retain water, making more concentrated urine.

In a person without diabetes, when they are thirsty or even dehydrated, the levels of the antidiuretic hormone increase. The kidneys will naturally reabsorb more water and release highly concentrated urine. Conversely, in a person with diabetes insipidus, two problems can occur related to the antidiuretic hormone – not enough being produced and an inability on behalf of the kidneys to properly respond to the antidiuretic hormone being created.

When there is not enough of the antidiuretic hormone being produced, this leads to a condition called central diabetes insipidus. When there is enough of the hormone being produced, but an inability for the kidneys to properly respond to it, this is called nephrogenic diabetes insipidus.

No matter which type of diabetes insipidus a person has, the end result is the same – the kidneys are not able to perform the task of conserving water, leading to diabetes insipidus. When an individual who has diabetes insipidus is dehydrated, the kidneys will continue to pass large quantities of diluted urine, leading to further complications.

In order to diagnose diabetes insipidus, doctors will measure the amounts of blood and urine over a period of several hours, as the patient is deprived of water and becomes increasingly more thirsty. Depending on the results of these tests, the patient may then be given an antidiuretic hormone substitute and monitored further to determine if the kidneys respond by producing concentrated urine, determining the diagnosis of diabetes insipidus.

Because the kidneys are still able to perform their main task – blood filtering – diabetes insipidus does not lead to kidney failure and/or dialysis. Due to the extreme levels of urination associated with diabetes insipidus, diagnosed individuals need to ensure constant consumption of water, particularly in hotter temperatures.

What Causes Diabetes?

As there are many different types of diabetes, each working in a different way, it is natural that the cause of each type is different. Here you will learn what doctors suspect causes each type of diabetes, as some of the situations can be quite difficult.

Causes of Type 1 Diabetes

Similar to many other diseases, doctors do not know exactly what causes Type 1 diabetes, or at least not every cause to the disease. It has been determined, however, that Type 1 diabetes can be passed down from generation to generation. Further, physicians have determine that there is an environmental factor, such as a virus or toxin – albeit they are not quite sure which one – that sets the immune system in action to attack the pancreas, destroying the beta cells, leaving them unable to produce sufficient amounts of insulin.

This leads doctors to classify Type 1 diabetes as an autoimmune disease, which can occur with others in its class, including hyperthyroidism that develops from Grave's disease and/or a condition known as vitiligo where patches of the skin show signs of decreased pigmentation.

Causes of Type 2 Diabetes

Although the most common causes of Type 2 diabetes is lack of physical activity and being overweight, they are not the only two factors that lead to this disease. Other factors include the nonexistent production of insulin by the pancreas or the production of very little insulin or when the body is insulin resistant, meaning the body does not know how to respond to the insulin that is produced.

As has been mentioned several times, the improper use or lack of insulin leads to large amounts of sugar being trapped in the bloodstream, as opposed to moving into the cells to be used for energy. This is what causes high blood sugar levels, thus causing diabetes, or in this case, Type 2 diabetes.

Causes of Gestational Diabetes

Gestational diabetes is a type of diabetes that results from pregnancy. During pregnancy the placenta – sack that holds the fetus during pregnancy and serves as a means of food and water – develops in the uterus. The placenta also produces a variety of hormones, some of which create problems for insulin to control blood sugar levels. When this happens, it is necessary for the mother's body to produce more insulin in order to maintain proper blood sugar levels. Unfortunately, during pregnancy the pancreas may not be able to produce enough insulin to maintain the proper blood sugar levels, resulting in gestational diabetes.

Causes of Prediabetes

In a nutshell, prediabetes is a result of insulin resistance, and if left untreated leads to Type 2 diabetes. Insulin resistance occurs when the body's cells no longer have the ability to respond to the insulin the body produces. In turn, this causes the pancreas to produce and secrete more insulin, leaving high levels of insulin in the blood. While this does not necessarily mean an individual has diabetes, it does mean they have prediabetes, or higher than normal blood sugar levels. Without treatment and over time, this can lead to Type 2 diabetes.

Causes of Diabetes Insipidus

The main underlying factor of diabetes insipidus is attributed two different problems associated with the antidiuretic hormone produced by the brain. When the brain does not produce enough antidiuretic hormone this is known as central diabetes insipidus. On the other hand, when the brain produces proper amount of the antidiuretic hormone but the kidney fails to respond, this is known as nephrogenic diabetes insipidus. Either way, the kidneys can no longer perform the task of water conservation, leading to excessive thirst and high levels of urine production, both of which can lead to electrolyte imbalances.

What Are the Symptoms Associated with Diabetes?

Similar to each type of diabetes having its own set of causes, the symptoms of the various types of diabetes can be different as well. It is important that anyone experiencing the symptoms associated with diabetes – no matter the type – speak with their physician to ensure they are diagnosed, treated and learn to properly manage their diabetes for a longer, healthier life free from complications caused by diabetes.

Symptoms of Type 1 Diabetes

Although subtle, the symptoms associated with Type 1 diabetes can become increasingly severe. This can include increased thirst and hunger, even after having just eaten, dry mouth and constant urination. Other individuals diagnosed with Type 1 diabetes have noticed nausea and vomiting, abdominal pain, unexplained weight loss, feeling tired or weak and infections, such as skin infections, urinary tract infections and vaginal infections.

In the event of an emergency associated with Type 1 diabetes, individuals may experience shaking and confusion, rapid breathing, abdominal pain and a fruity smelling breath. In rare cases, some patients have lost consciousness. If any of the above symptoms have been experienced, it is important to seek emergency medical care in order to be tested, diagnosed and treated for Type 1 diabetes.

Symptoms of Type 2 Diabetes

Because Type 2 diabetes can result in serious health complications, such as heart attack and stroke, it is important to know, understand and be aware of the associated symptoms. Similar to Type 1 diabetes, individuals may experience increased thirst, feeling hungry even after eating, dry mouth and frequent urination. Other symptoms of Type 2 diabetes include weight loss, feeling tired or weak, blurred vision and headaches. With rare cases, it is possible to experience a loss of consciousness. Talking with a healthcare provider is important to determine whether or not the symptoms experienced are a result of Type 2 diabetes.

Symptoms of Gestational Diabetes

Unfortunately, gestational diabetes does not present with any symptoms. This is why, when a woman is pregnant, the physician will order a glucose tolerance test somewhere around the 24th and 28th week of pregnancy to avoid complications during pregnancy, labor and delivery and ensure the mother and baby are healthy. However, there are some instances where, during pregnancy, a woman may discover/develop symptoms of diabetes she may never know she had. This can include increased levels of thirst, urination and hunger, as well as blurred vision. Because the first three symptoms are often signs of being pregnant as well, it is important that discussions with a physician are scheduled and the glucose tolerance test is taken.

Symptoms of Prediabetes

Symptoms of diabetes can be quite difficult to determine in some cases. This is particularly true with prediabetes, wherein technically there are no signs or symptoms associated with prediabetes. With that said, some individuals do experience some changes that send them to their physicians, where tests determine they do have prediabetes. This can include an increase in feeling thirsty, increased feeling of needing to urinate, blurred vision and in some cases, extreme fatigue.

Symptoms of Diabetes Insipidus

Diabetes insipidus has two levels of symptoms – one for the disease itself and another for resulting dehydration and fluid loss. First, individuals with undiagnosed diabetes insipidus will likely experience extreme levels of feeling thirsty and polyuria – extreme need for urination. Because these symptoms lead to dehydration, it is likely the individual will experience electrolyte imbalances. The symptoms associated with electrolyte imbalances, thus associated with diabetes insipidus are unexplained weakness and lethargy, muscle pains and irritability. Due to the severe nature of symptoms associated with diabetes insipidus, it is very important that anyone who experiences these symptoms speaks with a physician in order to gain control of their disease.

Treatment for Diabetes – What's the Plan?

While it may take some time to get medications right and working properly and will definitely take some determination and will to get better from the individual, diabetes is either manageable or treatable and in some cases, completely reversible. Because each type of diabetes is due to a different cause and has different symptoms, it only stands to reason that treatment methods are going to be different. Talking with a physician, monitoring blood sugar levels and following doctor's orders are only the beginning in the process to treating diabetes.

Treatment of Type 1 Diabetes

Although Type 1 diabetes does require lifelong treatment, monitoring blood sugar levels, changing eating habits and taking medication – typically insulin injections or wearing an insulin pump – people can enjoy a fulfilling life while treating their Type 1 diabetes. The biggest concern when treating Type 1 diabetes – or any type of diabetes for that matter – is maintaining blood sugar levels to keep them within normal limits.

Aside from self-testing blood sugar levels on a regular basis, individuals with Type 1 diabetes will need regularly scheduled visits with their physician in order to ensure no complications have begun, such as kidney, eye, heart, nerve and blood vessel issues.

As with any type of disease, a healthy diet and exercise plan can keep blood sugar levels maintained and reduce the risk of other complications associated with Type 1 diabetes, particularly those concerning the heart and blood vessels. It is also important for an individual with Type 1 diabetes to not smoke and not drink alcoholic beverages, especially if they are at risk for having low blood sugar levels.

Treatment of Type 2 Diabetes

Similar to Type 1 diabetes, treatment of Type 2 diabetes involves monitoring blood sugar levels, a healthy diet and exercise. However, because the most common cause of Type 2 diabetes is obesity, physicians may recommend different treatment patterns and goals. For instance, weight loss surgery, such as gastric bypass, is becoming increasingly more popular as a means for treatment. Individuals who use weight loss surgery as a means of treatment must be willing to make lifestyle changes, particularly when it comes to eating habits and increasing physical activity.

Other methods of treatment typically recommended by physicians include medication, either oral or non-insulin diabetes injections, as individuals with Type 2 diabetes often produce insulin on their own, whereas individuals with Type 1 diabetes do not. Metformin is the most commonly prescribed injectable medication used for treatment of Type 2 diabetes. Some examples of oral diabetes medications include sulfonylureas, biguanides, thiazolidinediones and meglitinides, to name a few. Depending on each individual situation, physicians will determine the best medication that is right for each patient diagnosed with Type 2 diabetes, and in some cases, a combination of two or more medications may be the right answer.

There are times where an individual diagnosed with Type 2 diabetes does need insulin injections. This will be determined through testing to see whether or not the body is making proper amounts of insulin. When taking insulin, or any diabetes medication, blood sugar levels need to be monitored on a daily basis and regular visits with the physician are necessary to ensure blood sugar levels are being maintained within normal limits.

Again, a healthy balanced diabetic diet and increasing physical activity are the simplest ways of helping to control blood sugar levels and preventing further complications. Furthermore, Type 2 diabetes is reversible – especially if the cause is related to obesity and talking with a physician is the first step in not only treating Type 2 diabetes but curing or reversing the disease.

Treatment of Gestational Diabetes

Because gestational diabetes only results due to hormonal changes in pregnant women, typical treatment methods only include following a well-balanced diabetic diet and adding exercise into the daily routine. However, if a woman at risk for developing diabetes prior to becoming pregnant, for instance, being overweight or having symptoms of diabetes, it is important to get tested before getting pregnant or as soon as pregnancy is confirmed. This will ensure proper treatment and better management during pregnancy to safeguard the mother and child from complications and possible birth defects.

Treatment of Prediabetes

Typically, there are no medications prescribed for individuals with prediabetes, as it is just a precursor to diabetes and not the disease. With that said, individuals with prediabetes need to be careful and follow certain physician recommendations in order to reverse prediabetes and prevent Type 2 diabetes from occurring.

This can be done in three easy steps – weight, diet, exercise. By monitoring weight and maintaining a healthy BMI based on height, weight and age, following a healthy balanced diet with an emphasis on diabetic healthy foods and becoming more active, any individual can stop prediabetes from turning into Type 2 diabetes.

Treatment of Diabetes Insipidus

Because diabetes insipidus causing extreme thirst and dehydration to the point of hospitalization, the main treatment regimen is drinking lots of fluids – maybe even more than one thinks is needed. Aside from that, there are other measures that can be taking depending on which type of diabetes insipidus an individual is diagnosed with.

For instance, someone diagnosed with central diabetes insipidus can replace missing antidiuretic hormone simply by taking a nasal spray known as vasopressin, or using the oral form of the medication. Conversely, individuals diagnosed with nephrogenic diabetes insipidus may have a more difficult time with treatment. This is mainly due to the fact that finding the cause of the nephrogenic diabetes insipidus can often be tricky. If it is found to be due to a different medication, typically ceasing to take the medication can reduce urination, thus treating the diabetes insipidus. Furthermore, there are some medications, such as indomethacin or diuretics, such as hydrochlorothiazide, that can improve symptoms associated with nephrogenic diabetes insipidus.

All in all, treatment of diabetes – no matter what the type – begins with managing blood sugar levels. The next step is to ensure these levels stay within normal ranges through a well-balanced diabetic diet, exercise and in some cases, medications. Talking with a physician about what treatment plan is right for each individual is definitely a key factor in managing, treating and in some cases, reversing diabetes.

Chapter 2 – Diabetes & Eating – What's Right & Wrong?

"What can I eat?," is one of the first questioned asked of physicians when they give the news that their patient has been diagnosed with diabetes. While this is a good question, it is not something that should make a diabetic feel restricted from eating the foods they like or deprived of having their favorite snack.

As will be discussed, there are certain foods a diabetic should and can eat and other foods they should avoid or limit the best they can. It is also important to gain knowledge of how much and how often a diabetic should eat in order to manage and treat their diabetes. The diabetic diet is not just some new diet to try out and then give up, but should be considered more of a new way of life.

Choosing Healthy Foods

In order to maintain healthy blood sugar levels choosing healthy foods is key. Everyone has heard the age-old story of eating fruits and vegetables, but there is so much more that goes into a healthy diabetic diet, albeit fruits and vegetables are a major part of it. A well-balanced diabetic diet is about choosing healthy foods from a wide variety of what's out there. However, because there are so many different foods, some claiming to be healthy, others known to be bad, choosing the right healthy foods for a diabetic diet can be difficult.

Fruits & Vegetables

Choosing fruits and vegetables adds many vitamins, minerals and fiber, but because they do contain carbohydrates, they need to be counted as part of the diabetic meal plan. However, there are some fruits and vegetables that are more suitable than others. For instance, when it comes to fruits, fresh, canned or frozen – those without any added sugars should be chosen. If canned fruits are the only type available, they need to be canned in juice or light syrup – never heavy syrup. Good fruit choices include apples, bananas, grapefruit, oranges, pineapples, grapes, strawberries and watermelon, to name a few.

Vegetables can be a bit more tricky, as some vegetables can be starchy, which are the types that should not be chosen. Non-starchy vegetables, or the good vegetables, include spinach, asparagus, green beans, cabbage, cauliflower, carrots, celery, eggplant and leeks. Similar to fruit, it is important to pay attention to what the vegetables are packaged in. When choosing canned or frozen vegetables, choose those that say no salt added or those that contain low sodium. Avoid vegetables packaged in sauces, as those tend to add unnecessary fats and sodium. If no other vegetables are available, rinse vegetables that are canned in sodium to remove as much as possible.

Now that there are options for the right fruits and vegetables, the next question is, how much fruits and vegetables should a diabetic individual consume on a daily basis. As a general rule, consuming 3-5 servings of vegetables per day can lead to better management of diabetes.

One serving of vegetables is approximately ½ cup of cooked vegetables or 1 cup of raw vegetables.

Portion sizes with fruits can be a little more difficult, as the serving size really depends on which fruit you choose. For example, when choosing fresh berries or melons, a serving size is between ¾ cup and 1 cup. For whole fresh fruits, or those canned or frozen, ½ cup is a typical serving size. Dried fruits are also a good choice, although not as fulfilling, and a serving size of raisins, for instance, is only 2 tablespoons.

Lean Meats

Enough about fruits and vegetables, what else is suitable for a diabetic diet? It is recommended that an individual with diabetes choose fish at least three times a week and lean cuts of meat – any that have the word "loin" in them are best. Examples of good fish to include in a diabetic diet are catfish, flounder, orange roughy, salmon, tilapia and tuna. Good meat choices include pork tenderloin, veal loin and sirloin steak. When it comes to poultry, always choose skinless chicken and turkey, as opposed to those with skin on.

A general rule when choosing proper portions of meats is choosing a piece that is somewhere between 2 and 5 ounces. Avoid those with breading, as they add unnecessary carbohydrates. Reading food labels can really help with making the right choices and will provide pertinent information, such as the weight of the meat choice.

Non-Fat Dairy

Dairy is next on the list and choosing non-fat dairy products is the best choice. This can include items like skim milk, non-fat cheese and non-fat yogurts. Soymilk is a good alternative to regular dairy products, but needs to be unflavored. Choose plain yogurts, as opposed to those with fruit added in. Fresh fruits can be added in to plain yogurt, but remember to count them as part of the overall diabetic plan.

A good tip when it comes to switching over to non-fat dairy products is to take small steps. If whole milk has been the choice in the household, first switch to 2% and then work down to 1% and then move on to skim milk. This will help individuals get used to the taste and texture of the different percentages, while still cutting back unnecessary calories and fat with each step. When it comes to portion sizes, approximately 1 cup, or 8 ounces, of milk or 2/3 cup of yogurt is the standard size.

Understanding Carbohydrates

Carbohydrates are one of the top food items to be the first thing kicked out of every diet. While it is important to limit carbohydrates, understanding them and knowing when to eat them and how much to eat is a better option, particularly if pasta and bread are among the favorites in foods consumed before being diagnosed with diabetes.

It is important to know that there are three main types of carbohydrates – starches (complex carbohydrates), sugars and fiber. When it comes to choosing the right carbohydrates, it really comes down to knowing how to read the food labels. The phrase "total carbohydrates" appears on food labels, contains all three types and should be the one used to calculate carbohydrate intake on the diabetic diet.

Starch

Limiting foods high in starch is the first step. Surprisingly, there are quite a few vegetables that can be knocked of the list – peas, lima beans, corn and potatoes. While there are some dried beans that are good for you, other such as pinto beans, black-eyed peas and kidney beans also tend to have a high starch content.

There are also some grains with high starch that should be limited also, including rice, barley and oats. However, grains can actually be broken into two different categories – whole grains and refined grains – meaning there are some that can be included in the diabetic diet plan. It makes sense that whole grains are the ones that should be chosen, but understanding why can help make the decision.

Each grain contains three components – bran, germ and endosperm. Bran is the hard outer shell of the grain and provides the most fiber, minerals and B vitamins. The next layer is germ, which provides essential nutrients such as vitamin E and fatty acids. The last layer is the center or endosperm, which is the starch part.

The term "whole grain" means that the food is made with all three parts of the grain, not just the endosperm, which is all that can be found in refined grain foods. Choosing whole grain foods, such as whole grain pasta, means that you get all the vitamins, minerals and nutrients a grain has to offer, not just the unhealthy starch.

Sugar

The next type of carbohydrate is sugar, of which there are two types – naturally occurring sugars and added sugars. Naturally occurring sugars are contained in fruit and milk, while added sugars are just that – added at the time the foods are processed and packaged, such as the heavy syrup that is added to many canned fruits.

With sugars it is important to read the label, where the total sugar will be a combination of both natural and added sugars. While that seems simple to understand, there are a few different names for sugar – whether natural or added – that an individual planning a diabetic diet needs to be aware of.

In fact, sugar can be called more than ten different things but is still sugar. Sugar is often referred to as brown sugar, molasses, beet sugar, honey, powdered sugar, syrup – maple, high-fructose corn, sugar cane – and agave nectar. Sometimes, the chemical name for sugar is listed – sucrose – and can also be found in other terms with the "ose" ending, such as fructose, fruit syrup and lactose or the sugar found in milk. No matter which way sugar is listed on a food label, it's still sugar and needs to be limited when planning a diabetic diet.

Fiber

Fiber is the third type of carbohydrate and comes only from plant foods and will not be found in animal products, including eggs, meat, fish, poultry or milk. Although fiber is very good for any individual, it is not digested as it passes through the intestines. However, fiber is still an important part of digestive health, helping to keep bowel movements regular and offering a feeling of being full longer.

Eating a diet high in fiber has also been attributed to lowering cholesterol levels. Unfortunately, most adults only take in about half of the suggested daily intake of approximately 25-30 grams of fiber daily. Reaching this high level of fiber intake can be quite difficult, even though it is recommended. On the other hand, any increase in fiber can be beneficial on any diet, including the diabetic diet plan.

In order to increase dietary fiber intake, physicians recommend eating beans and legumes, particularly black beans, pinto beans, kidney beans, white bean and chickpeas. Other foods that serve as a good source of fiber include fruits and vegetables with edible skin or edible seeds, such as apples, beans and berries. Whole grains, including whole-wheat pasta and whole grain cereals that contain more than 3 grams of dietary fiber are also excellent sources of fiber. For a light snack, nuts, such as peanuts, almonds and walnuts also provide high amounts of fiber, but need to be consumed in small quantities, as they also have high calories.

Choosing good sources of fiber is done simply by looking at the amount of dietary fiber. It is recommended that foods with 2.5 - 4.9 grams of fiber per serving are the ones that should be chosen. Further, although there are supplements that can be taken to increase fiber, it is better to eat foods that are rich in fiber, as those will provide more nutritional benefit that a supplement. A word to the wise however, increase daily fiber in small steps and drink plenty of water in order to avoid stomach irritation and constipation.

Learn the Diabetes Super Foods

Everyday someone somewhere comes out with a new list of foods that should be eaten in order to jump-start a diet plan. The question comes to mind, however, do any of those foods fit in with a diabetic diet plan? The answer is yes, here are is a list of the top ten foods that are not only contain a low glycemic index, but also provide important nutrients, such as calcium, fiber, potassium, magnesium and vitamins A, C and E.

1. Beans – First on the list is one that keeps popping up in almost every section of the diabetic diet plan – beans. It does not matter if a person prefers one kind to another, there is no other food that provides so much nutrition in one little bean. Beans are not only high in fiber, providing about 1/3 of your needed fiber intake per day, but are full of magnesium and potassium as well. Excellent sources of these nutrients can be found in navy beans, black beans, pinto beans and kidney beans.

2. Dark Green Leafy Vegetables – Choosing dark leafy green vegetables is a no-brainer when it comes to get more vitamins and minerals without all the calories. This can include kale, collard greens and spinach.

3. Citrus Fruit – The next item on the list of diabetic top ten super foods to be aware of are citrus fruits, such as grapefruit, limes, lemons and oranges. They offer up not only vitamin C, but fiber as well.

4. Sweet Potatoes – Although a starchy vegetable, sweet potatoes are full of fiber and vitamin A. This diabetic super food can be eaten in place of a white potato.

5. Berries – Not only are all berries – whether you choose blueberries, blackberries or strawberries – full of fiber and vitamins, but they also provide a high amount of antioxidants. To satisfy every sweet tooth satisfied, layer non-fat yogurt and berries for a delicious dessert.

6. Tomatoes – Although best in the summer when they come fresh from the garden, tomatoes are an excellent source of vitamin E, vitamin C and iron. This diabetic super food can be eaten just about any way – raw or in sauce and the nutritional benefit is still there.

7. Omega-3 Fatty Acid Rich Fish – The top fish in this category is salmon, but only the variety that is not breaded and fried. Choose grilled salmon to turn this fish into a diabetic super food.

8. Whole Grains – Making the list yet again is whole grains – offering a large quantity of fiber, vitamins, minerals, and so much more – this super food needs to be added to every diabetic diet.

9. Nuts & Seeds – Nuts do provide healthy fats and are excellent sources of magnesium and fiber. In addition, walnuts and flax seeds offer a good amount of omega-3 fatty acids as well.

10. Fat-Free Milk & Yogurt – Not only does dairy build healthy teeth and strong bones, but is the major source of vitamin D, which has been on just about every physician's watch list the last few years.

Limit Sugar & Desserts

Many people believe that sugar is what causes diabetes, even though this is not entirely true. What people don't know about sugar and diabetes is that for individuals with Type 1 diabetes, the problem is genetic – not caused by sugar. For individuals with Type 2 diabetes, the main cause is being overweight, which sugar attributes to but is not solely responsible for.

With that said, however, the amount of sugar consumed by individuals with diabetes does need to be monitored. This is not to say that a diabetic is banned from ever eating sweets again, but it does mean that they need to be limited – saved for special occasions. It is more important for a diabetic person's body to have the vital nutrients it receives from other foods before it receives sugars in desserts.

As long as a proper diabetic diet plan is in place, a diabetic can have their cake and eat it too – once in a while. Particularly, this deals with cutting back on other high sugar foods – whether natural or not – and cutting back on foods high in carbohydrates to allow room for dessert, literally.

Choose the Right Fats

One food that is very difficult for anyone to get a grasp on what is right and what is wrong is fats, because yes, there are some good fats that should be included as part of a healthy, well-balance diabetic meal plan – or any meal plan for that matter. It is important to understand what the different types of fats are and whether or not they plan a negative or positive role in overall health.

The good fats, or unsaturated fats, as they are so called have been linked with lowering a person's risk of developing heart disease. On the other hand, the bad fats, such as saturated fats and trans fats do the opposite by increasing the risk of heart disease. Although all fats typically contain a high amount of calories, by choosing the right ones in moderation, they can add not only flavor, but nutritional benefits as well.

Good Fats

Whether the label says polyunsaturated or monounsaturated or even omega-3, these are all the good fats. If a recipe calls for oil, try and substitute using a vegetable oil, such as olive, cottonseed, grape seed, safflower or sunflower, to name a few. When it comes to spreading on the "good stuff" choose mayonnaise or trans-fat-free margarine or margarines made with plant sterols.

There are some foods that contain good fats, which can be eaten on a diabetic diet, such as avocado, olives, and a variety of nuts, including pecans, cashews, walnuts and pistachios. However, because these do still contain fat, they should be consumed in limited quantities.

Bad Fats

As was already discussed, but important enough to mention again, saturated and trans fats are indeed the bad fats. Both of these types of fats are not only loaded with calories, but can increase the risk of developing heart disease and/or stroke. For cooking oils, any individual and particularly a diabetic, should avoid coconut oil, lard, palm oil and shortening. All of these contain bad fats.

Spreads that contain bad fats include butter and margarine that contains trans fats, sour cream and cream cheese. Other foods that make the list of bad fat content are bacon, coconut, cream, salt pork and chitterlings. It is important for a diabetic to try and completely remove these types of foods from their everyday diet, or at least cut back as much as possible to lower the risk of heart disease, stroke and in order to treat and reduce the effects of diabetes on the body.

Artifical Sweeteners – Are They Really Better?

For years that has been controversy over whether or not artificial sweeteners – particularly those in the sugar alcohol family – are better than regular sugar. While some information will be reported here, the debate is still up in the air, as there are advantages and disadvantages to consuming sugar alcohols over regular sugar.

First and foremost, it is important to note that sugar alcohols, despite their name, do not actually contain alcohol. The next thing is explaining what exactly sugar alcohols are then, if they're not alcohol. They are reduced-calorie sweeteners that not only provide less calories that regular sugar, but also have a smaller impact on blood sugar levels than other carbohydrates. Sugar alcohols go by a variety of different chemical names, including glycerin, isomalt, mannitol and sorbitol.

Advantages

The simplest way to discuss the advantages of reduced-calorie sweeteners is just that – they have less calories. Therefore, if an individual is trying to prevent weight gain or to lose weight, low-calories sweeteners definitely have the upper hand. Many times, reduced-calorie sweeteners, such as sugar alcohols, also have fewer carbohydrates, thus having less effect on blood sugar levels, making them easier to maintain.

Disadvantages

With that said, however, there are some disadvantages, particularly the fact that foods produced with reduced-calorie sweeteners typically contain more fats and not the good ones. Many prepackaged baked goods that boast the title of being made with a particular sugar alcohol, more than likely contains saturated fats and trans fats that its regular sugar counterpart may not have. These bad fats are used to make up for the loss of flavor from using real sugar. Might not be so bad, except for they increase the risk of heart disease and stroke, which nobody wants.

Further, foods made with reduced-calorie sweeteners, particularly sugar alcohols, often have a laxative effect or can produce other negative gastric symptoms. This is particularly true from children, who are more affected by sugar alcohols than adults. In addition, there are many instances where the sugar-free product actually costs more than the product made with regular sugar.

Although there are some benefits to choosing sugar alcohol sweeteners, many people choose to eat the foods with regular sugar instead. However, they reduce their potion sizes, to compensate for the negative effects that regular sugar can have on them, particularly those individuals who have been diagnosed with diabetes.

What to Eat – Summary

There are a lot of foods that a diabetic individual should eat, but what it really boils down to is a well-balanced healthy diet, full of foods that are low in fat and high in protein, vitamins and minerals. The basics include the following steps:

1: Eat 3-5 servings each of fruits and vegetables – fresh are better than canned or frozen, when available.

2: Choose lean cuts of meat, such as those with the word "loin" in them, with portions somewhere between 2 and 5 ounces.

3: Choose non-fat dairy products, such as skim milk and non-fat plain yogurt.

4: Choose foods that are high in dietary fiber to reduce cholesterol levels and to help keep your digestive system regular. Look for whole grain breads, cereals and pastas.

5: Become familiar with the diabetes super foods and be sure to include them in your diabetic diet meal plan.

6: Choose the good fats, such as those made from vegetable or plant products or that are labeled polyunsaturated, monounsaturated or omega-3 fatty acids.

What to Avoid - Summary

While nobody wants to hear about foods they need to avoid, there are some that really should be left out of a diabetic diet plan. Not only do these foods offer little to no nutritional value but the negative effects that have on one's health, particularly a diabetic, is not worth having that little bit of something extra. Remembering what types of foods to avoid can be simple by following the guidelines below:

1. Avoid starchy vegetables, as they have unnecessary carbohydrates and there are many alternative vegetable choices. Pass over the canned fruit that is packaged in heavy syrup and the vegetables prepared in sauces.

2. Say no to meats that have the skin on, are breaded and/or deep fat fried.

3. Avoid full fat dairy and yogurt that has fruit added in. Add your own fresh fruit instead.

4. Limit starches by choosing whole grains and avoid added sugars, eating only what's found naturally in foods.

5. Limit sugars and desserts and plan ahead for special occasions, such as wanting a slice of birthday cake or grandma's apple pie.

6. Forget about bad fats – the saturated and trans fats – these can be done without.

Following these easy guidelines will put you on the right track to choosing the right foods, planning meals, putting you on the right road to managing your diabetes.

Chapter 3 – Diabetic Meal Plan

Chapter 1 described the different types of diabetes, including what they are, the symptoms, the causes and some treatment methods. The focus of Chapter 2 was what types of foods diabetics should and shouldn't eat. Now, in this chapter you will discover how to apply all of the information you have just read about to your daily routine. There will be meal plans for breakfast, lunch, dinner and snacks to get you through the day for one week. There will also be alternative choice suggestions in case there is something on the "menu" that doesn't fancy your taste buds.

The Basics

In order to plan meals, you will want to follow the guidelines, tips and information you found in Chapter 2. It is particularly important to pay attention to carbohydrate and calorie intake, trying to keep yourself around 1,600 calories per day with no more than 220 grams of carbohydrates per day. It is also important to drink lots of water. In fact, it is recommended that with each meal you drink two eight-ounce glasses. Here are a few sample meal plans for breakfast, lunch and dinner that should get you through your first week, maybe two, depending on how many of the meal options you like. With that said, each meal can be altered to your liking, but be sure and stick to the diabetic meal plan guidelines when making changes, limiting yourself to two healthy snacks per day.

Meal Plan Examples

WEEK 1

DAY 1

BREAKFAST	LUNCH	DINNER	SNACKS
1 slice whole wheat toast 1 egg poached ½ cup skim milk ½ small banana	1 cup vegetable soup w/ 5 low-sodium crackers 1 turkey sandwich made from 2 slices whole wheat bread, 1 ounce skinless turkey and 1 ounce low-fat cheese w/ 1 teaspoon mayonnaise 1 small apple	4-ounce grilled chicken breast w/herbs ½ cup brown rice ½ cup steamed carrots 1 small whole grain dinner roll 1 cup mixed greens salad w/ 2 tablespoons non-fat dressing 1 slice broiled pineapple	1 cup grapes ½ cup sugar free chocolate pudding

DAY 2

BREAKFAST	LUNCH	DINNER	SNACKS
1 scrambled egg 1 slice whole wheat toast 1 cup fresh strawberries ½ cup skim milk	Small mixed greens w/grapes & feta cheese salad 1 cup bean soup w/greens 5 low-sodium crackers	4-ounce portion of turkey cutlet broiled w/sage & lemon Warm red cabbage salad ½ cup steamed broccoli Baked sweet potato ½ cup skim milk	1 cup grapes 1 slice non-fat cheese

DAY 3

BREAKFAST	LUNCH	DINNER	SNACKS
1 slice baked cheese & asparagus frittata 1 cup skim milk 1 small orange	1 cup tomato soup 1 grilled cheese sandwich made w/ 2 slices whole wheat bread and 1 slice low-fat cheese 1 cup melon cubes	Grilled pork tenderloin marinated in rosemary & apples Small tossed salad w/ 2 tablespoons non-fat dressing ½ cup brown rice	1 small apple 1 slice non-fat cheese

DAY 4

BREAKFAST	LUNCH	DINNER	SNACKS
1 slice whole wheat toast 1 cup low-fat plain yogurt 1 cup fresh strawberries ½ cup skim milk	1 cup pea soup	1 slice sausage, mushroom & spinach lasagna 1 cup sliced tomato salad ½ cup steamed asparagus ½ cup apricot halves	1 banana sliced 5 low-sodium crackers

DAY 5

BREAKFAST	LUNCH	DINNER	SNACKS
1 whole grain berry muffin 1 cup skim milk 1 cup cubed melon	2 chicken tacos on whole wheat tortillas with ½ ounce low-fat cheese each, lettuce & pico de gallo 1 cup grapes	Small spinach salad w/ fat-free vinaigrette dressing 4-ounce grilled fish (your choice) w/lemon & herbs ½ cup brown rice ½ cup fresh berries & non-fat yogurt	1 slice non-fat cheese 1 cup celery sticks

DAY 6

BREAKFAST	LUNCH	DINNER	SNACKS
2 small whole wheat blueberry pancakes 1 cup non-fat yogurt ½ cup skim milk	1 turkey burger w/honey mustard on whole wheat bun 1 cup broccoli slaw ½ cup skim milk 1 cup strawberries	4-ounce grilled sirloin steak w/mushrooms & onions 1 cup steamed cauliflower 1 small slice angel food cake	1/2 cup frozen strawberry yogurt 5 low-sodium crackers

DAY 7

BREAKFAST	LUNCH	DINNER	SNACKS
1 slice whole wheat toast 1 egg scrambled ½ grapefruit 1 cup skim milk	1 slice chicken pot pie Small tossed salad w/ 2 tablespoons non-fat dressing ½ cup non-fat yogurt	1 cup gnocchi w/crushed tomatoes ½ cup steamed broccoli ½ cup brown rice ½ cup apricot halves	1 cup celery sticks 1 slice non-fat cheese

WEEK 2

DAY 8

BREAKFAST	LUNCH	DINNER	SNACKS
1 cup oatmeal w/1/2 cup fresh berries 1 slice whole wheat toast 1 cup skim milk	1 cup wedding soup 5 low-sodium crackers 1 cup melon cubes	4-ounce grilled sirloin steak ½ cup baked sweet potato fries ½ cup grilled asparagus 1 cup pineapple	1 cup raw carrots ½ banana

DAY 9

BREAKFAST	LUNCH	DINNER	SNACKS
1 cup non-fat yogurt	1 cup tuna & white bean salad	4-ounce slice garlic-roasted pork loin	1 cup blueberries
1 slice whole wheat toast	½ whole wheat pita	1 cup shredded carrots	1 slice non-fat cheese
1 small orange	½ cup skim milk	1 cup cucumber salad	
½ cup skim milk	1 small apple	1 cup fresh raspberries	

DAY 10

BREAKFAST	LUNCH	DINNER	SNACKS
1 egg poached 1 slice whole wheat toast 1 cup skim milk ½ cup fresh berries	1 turkey & tomato Panini on whole wheat bread w/1 ounce cheese 1 cup skim milk ½ banana	4-ounce broiled white fish w/lemon & herbs 1 cup steamed vegetable ribbons ½ cup brown rice 1 small slice angel food cake	1 banana 5 low-sodium crackers

DAY 11

BREAKFAST	LUNCH	DINNER	SNACKS
1 banana bran muffin ½ grapefruit 1 cup skim milk	1 cup shrimp cobb salad ½ whole wheat pita 1 cup skim milk	4-ounce grilled chicken breast with salsa ½ cup steamed carrots ½ cup couscous 1 cup blueberries	1 cup cubed melon 1 slice non-fat cheese

DAY 12

BREAKFAST	LUNCH	DINNER	SNACKS
1 cup oatmeal	1 cranberry & herb turkey burger	1 cup whole wheat pasta w/roasted vegetables	1 slice broiled pineapple
¼ cup cottage cheese			5 low-sodium crackers
½ small peach	1 ounce non-fat cheese	1 cup cucumber salad	
1 cup skim milk	1 cup spinach salad w/mushrooms, shredded carrots & non-fat vinaigrette	½ cup apricot halves	

DAY 13

BREAKFAST	LUNCH	DINNER	SNACKS
1 cup non-fat plain yogurt ½ cup fresh berries 1 slice whole wheat toast 1 cup skim milk	1 cup romaine salad w/ 4-ounce grilled chicken & apricots ½ whole wheat pita	4-ounce broiled white fish w/oranges & pecans ½ cup roasted broccoli w/lemon ½ cup brown rice 1 cup cubed melon	1 slice non-fat cheese 1 small apple

DAY 14

BREAKFAST	LUNCH	DINNER	SNACKS
1 egg poached 1 slice whole wheat toast 1 small orange ½ cup skim milk	½ cup fresh tuna salad on whole wheat bread 1 cup strawberries ½ cup skim milk	4-ounce pork medallions w/cranberries ½ cup steamed carrots 1 cup spinach salad w/grapes & feta 1 small whole wheat dinner roll ½ cup sliced pears	1 cup grapes 1 slice non-fat cheese

    Now that you have some idea of what a couple of weeks of eating for yourself might be, you can begin your well-balanced healthy diabetic diet without stressing over what to cook and how much is the right portion. If at any time you are concerned about your diabetic meal plan, it's a good idea to talk to your physician or a nutritional consultant at your doctor's office. They will be able to point you in the right direction with any questions you have regarding your diabetic meal planning process, from whether or not a certain food is a good idea to how often you are able to treat yourself to something special.

    It is also an excellent idea to plan your meals ahead of time, such as when you're planning your grocery shopping trip. If you have everything laid out before heading to the store, you will be able to prepare a grocery list of the essential items you will need for 1-2 weeks. This way, you will not end up filling your grocery cart full of things you don't need, as you already have a plan. Further, it's recommended that you never, ever go to the grocery store hungry. This causes impulse decisions, which are typically poor, where you end up putting unhealthy food and snack items into your cart. Try and plan your grocery trip after breakfast or lunch, as these are times when most people have the most energy and focus to stick to their planned grocery list, avoiding unnecessary healthy items.

Chapter 4 – Diabetic Diet Q&A

You've read all there is to read about diabetes general information, have prepared your meal plan for the next two weeks and are ready to hit the grocery store. Nevertheless, before you do, you still have a few questions that haven't been answered. Here in Chapter 4, you will find a lot of topics that diabetics are often concerned with when it comes to the diabetic diet planning process. Some questions may or may not pertain to you. In this section, it's fine if you only read the questions and answers that are pertinent to your particular situation, but feel free to read all question topics. The information is here for you to learn and that's what this book is all about.

Preventing Diabetes with Diabetic Diet – Can it be done?

Many people have often asked the question can diabetes be prevented simply by following a diabetic diet. The answer to this question is both yes and no. Following a diabetic diet will not prevent someone from developing Type 1 diabetes, but can prevent Type 2 diabetes and/or gestational diabetes.

As you read in Chapter 1, Type 1 diabetes is genetic, developing early in life, although typically not diagnosed until the teenage years. However, following a diabetic diet plan can be beneficial for someone with Type 1 diabetes, in that they will be able to maintain healthy blood sugar levels.

On the other hand, because Type 2 diabetes is not genetic, and typically caused by obesity, which can be heredity due to a child mimicking their parents' habits, following a diabetic diet can prevent this form of diabetes.

Further, gestational diabetes typically develops in women who are overweight prior to becoming pregnant. Therefore, following a diabetic diet plan will help you lose weight, increase overall healthiness, thus preventing the risk of developing diabetes.

Diabetic Diet for the Whole Family – Is it safe?

Trying to figure out what to have for dinner is never an easier task. Now that someone in the house has been diagnosed with diabetes, the challenge just got harder, right? Wrong, by following the diabetic diet guidelines in the previous chapters and taking from the sample menus, planning couldn't be easier. Wait, what about everyone else? Can everybody in the family eat the foods on a diabetic meal plan?

In general, a diabetic diet plan is really just a well-balanced, well-thought out, nutritious set of meals and snacks that any individual can follow to lead a healthy life. It is a perfect balance of natural sweets from fruits, lots of protein from dairy, meat and eggs, all the vitamins and minerals you could ask for without one thing – the unnecessary calories and carbohydrates. Thus, the diabetic diet is perfect for anyone who cares about health and wellness and wants to live a full and happy life.

Diabetic Diet for Teens & Picky Eaters – Is there such a thing?

Having a teenager, or younger child, diagnosed with diabetes can make planning a diabetic diet more difficult, particularly if he/she is a picky eater. Having said that, your child is going to do what you do, so if you change your eating habits, avoid making poor choices at the grocery store, your child will have no other choice but to eat fruits, vegetables, whole grains.

Yes, they may go hungry for the first couple of days, maybe even a week, but eventually they will give in and start trying some of the new healthy foods you are now purchasing. Keeping snacks away from them, such as chips, candy and soda is a great place to start. This isn't to say that they can never have a "treat" but their cravings can be found in healthy foods.

For kids, eating is a matter of convenience. Grabbing a bag of chips or a candy bar is convenient – change this – make fruits and vegetables convenient for them by having them cleaned, peeled and in bit size pieces perfect for snacking or having for dessert after dinner.

If you still cannot get your child to eat fruits and vegetables, try sneaking them into their diet. There are lots of recipes available via the web or library that offer different tips on adding both fruits and vegetables to your child's diet. For instance, if your child loves macaroni and cheese, ditch the box idea and make it from scratch. Puree up some carrots, use non-fat cheese and whole grain pasta. Because the carrots are orange – and really don't change the flavor – you child will be eating carrots – a vegetable – without even knowing it. You can sometimes sneak broccoli into the mix – in the chopped up steamed variety – and because is covered in gooey non-fat cheese, your child just might eat it.

You can also sneak vegetables into spaghetti sauce and cauliflower into mashed potatoes, again, by pureeing them. Other great "sneaky" food tips include using applesauce in a recipe that calls for oil – this adds great moisture – and you can avoid the additional preservatives by cooking and pureeing your own apples.

Smoothies are a great way of incorporating fruits and vegetables into your child's diet. They feel like they're getting a treat – especially if they get to use a straw – but smoothies are full of vitamins, minerals, fruits and vegetables. You can keep calories and carbohydrates down by using non-fat milk or non-fat yogurt and fresh fruits and vegetables, such as strawberries, bananas and vegetables that puree up nicely, such as carrots.

Most kids thoroughly enjoy French fries, albeit not a good side dish. However, if you use sweet potatoes cut into French fry-style strips and bake them, you are offering a better choice of one of your child's favorite foods. Pizza is another – make homemade pizza using whole wheat crust (healthy grain), crushed tomatoes or tomato sauce (vegetable), non-fat cheese, lean meats, such as turkey pepperoni, and vegetables – mushrooms, peppers, onions, etc. It seems when vegetables are placed on pizza, kids don't really think of them as vegetables. Pineapple also makes a great addition to pizza, but is sometimes a little harder for kids to grasp, especially when many adults don't choose it.

So you see, there are many ways of offering kids healthy choices, even if you have to sneak them. However, research has found that kids will eat more fruits and vegetables when not pressured, but offered the options as opposed to other unhealthy choices, like chips, candy, cakes, etc. Try it out, you never know what your kid will eat until it's offered to them!

Diabetic Meal Plan on the Go – What if I travel a lot?

For most people, travelling is a way of getting out of your ordinary life, ignoring emails, phone calls and forgetting you even have a job. It's a way to toss out your daily routine and have some fun. For others, travelling is part of work and something they do often. Either way, one routine you cannot let go of while traveling, if you're a diabetic, is your diet. Although managing diabetes during travel can be slightly more difficult, due to meals not prepared at home and changes in physical activity, planning ahead can really simplify things.

There are a few things you need to remember in order to manage your diabetes on the go. First and foremost, always pack double the amount of medication and supplies you think you will need, as you may experience travel delays, or if traveling for work, they may ask you to stay longer. It is also important to always have snacks, such as nuts and dried fruit, for times when your blood sugar levels may drop.

Secondly, prepare yourself for the specific type of traveling you will be doing. If you are traveling via the roadways, you can pack a cooler with foods that are hard to find on the road, such as fresh fruits, vegetables and yogurt. Always have a couple bottles of water with you whenever possible in order to keep yourself hydrated. If traveling by airplane, make sure to pack a small, healthy meal you can eat on the plane, if one is not provided by the airline.

Make sure you check your blood sugar levels often, as the food you eat, the lack of activity and changes in time zones can really change them. You should also keep to your normal exercise routine, as much as possible, aiming for at least 150 minutes of physical activity per week.

Lastly, because you will likely be dining at restaurants and diners, not preparing your own meals, you will need to make wise choices when ordering foods. Always have a glass of water with each meal, remember to have more vegetables on your plate than anything else – preferably not basted in butter or sauces, and be sure to include fruit, dairy and a small portion of lean meat. Remember, avoid fried foods and refined grains as much as possible and you will be on the right track to managing your diabetes while traveling and dining out.

Combining Gluten Free & Diabetic Meals

Individuals who have diabetes have to be careful of what they eat, how often and how much. This is even more important when that person has a coexisting condition, such as celiac disease. Celiac disease revolves around a particularly protein – gluten – which is found mostly in grains, such as barley, wheat, rye and some varieties of oats, in which individuals with celiac disease need to avoid these foods in order to prevent their small intestine being attacked by their immune system.

While each diet plan has its challenges, many feel that putting the two together can create a whole world of trouble – as far as planning, preparing and being satisfied from meals. However, by following a few simple guidelines, each disease can be managed side-by-side without problems.

For both, the main focus is a small portion of lean protein that is either baked, broiled or grilled with no breading, steamed or grilled vegetables, a serving of fruit and a small serving of brown rice for each meal. With the increasing awareness of celiac disease, many grocery stores are now carrying gluten-free product options, which are also sufficient for individuals with diabetes. There are even different types of gluten-free bread that is great for making a lean turkey sandwich for lunch.

However, you will still need to monitor blood sugar levels, of course, and be cautious of the amount of calories and carbohydrates you are consuming. You should never assume that gluten-free products have the same calorie and carbohydrate counts as other products you have purchased in the past. There are times when you will find that some gluten-free products have more than what you were used to and will need to adjust the rest of your meal to accommodate for the excess calories and carbohydrates. All in all, managing diabetes and celiac disease together can be accomplished with a little determination and slightly more effort, particularly when it comes to reading labels.

What is the Difference Between the Diabetic Diet & the Glycemic Index Diet?

Many people with diabetes have likely heard the term "glycemic index," but what does this mean and what's the difference between the glycemic index and a diabetic meal plan? The answer is simple, really – they have the ability to work together to manage diabetes. The glycemic index is a tool used to determine whether or not a food you choose is appropriate for a diabetic diet.

The glycemic index categorizes foods that contain carbohydrates depending on their effect on your blood sugar levels. Foods that increase your blood sugar rapidly and to higher levels, are considered to be foods that have a high glycemic index. Conversely, foods that slowly increase blood sugar levels, but not as high are considered to be low glycemic index foods.

Unfortunately, following a glycemic index diet or guide is not really all that simple. In fact, most foods, particularly those that are prepackaged, do not have a glycemic index rating on the label, making it difficult to determine where foods fall on the glycemic index.

There are some positives and negatives to using the glycemic index. On the upside, it can help lower blood sugar levels, keep them regulated, possibly reduce the need for medication to manage your diabetes and it can help control your appetite, thus managing your weight as well. On the downside, the foods listed on the glycemic index are ranked individually, not when prepared together, which can affect how your blood sugar levels change. Also, there are situations where the way a food impacts blood sugar levels is altered depending on how the food is prepared, which again, the glycemic index does not account for. Lastly, the glycemic index does not categorize and rank foods according to their nutrition content, meaning foods that are high in sugar, calories and/or saturated fat can be ranked low, and it only focuses on those that contain carbohydrates.

However, choosing the foods that you already know are "safe" for a diabetic, such as foods high in fiber, vegetables and fruits, you can be certain that your blood sugar levels will be controlled more often. If you are interested in using the glycemic index, it is a good suggestion to talk to your physician or a dietician to learn more about using the glycemic index as a tool for managing your diabetes.

What Role Does Exercise Play in Diabetes Management?

Physical activity, or exercise as it is often called, plays a major role in keeping individuals – with or without diabetes – healthy. Over the years research has been conducted on the effects of exercise on the body as a whole, and has been accredited to correcting and/or preventing many negative health risks.

Research has discovered that exercising, or participating in physical activity, a minimum of 30 minutes per day can lower blood pressure, blood sugar levels, bad cholesterol and body fat. It has been known to increase good cholesterol levels, boost energy levels and reduce stress levels, making for an overall happy individual. Exercising is a way to keep your heart in proper working fashion, increase bone strength and joint flexibility and has been known to improve your body's natural ability to make proper use of the insulin it produces.

Even though exercise has such a positive impact on healthy, many people still elect not to do it. This is often because they think of exercise as joining a gym, or running a mile through the park or on a treadmill. Although those are forms of exercise, physical activity comes in many different shapes and forms.

In fact, playing with your kids or walking around your house while talking on the phone counts as physical activity. Other examples of physical activity that can increase the control you have over your diabetes while decreasing your risk for further health complications includes walking your dog and doing yard work, such as mowing the law (with a push mower, of course), weeding the garden or raking leaves.

Many physicians count daily chores, such as cleaning your house, washing your car and doing laundry – especially if stairs are involved – as forms of physical activity. Parking your car farther away from the grocery store counts as physical activity.

If you enjoy walking and/or shopping, check out your local mall to find out when their morning walkers show up to do just that – walk around the mall without the traffic of shoppers. Typically, they will follow a certain path, but it is a great place to walk, as you are in out of the weather and you see something different around every corner. You can even stick around once the shops open and buy yourself some new clothes because, let's face it, after all that walking, you're bound to lose a few pounds.

Remember, no matter what you're doing, whether you're standing in the kitchen cooking supper, waiting for the water to boil, do a little dance, walk back and forth. The biggest thing to remember is just move! That's all physical activity and "exercise" are, just fancy names for movement, which everybody is capable of.

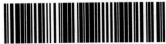